Special dedication

I whole heartedly dedicate this book to The Holy Trinity, who has been my guide and source of strength during those 60 days. They made sure I heard that small still voice every single day. Their wish is to see this program change your life.

******

Great dedications to my son Jacky-Junior and my daughter Maryne Sydney, for always being there to add some flavor and fun in my day to day life.

******

Another dedication to my sister Catherine and my niece Skyla, not only for their great support through the whole journey of this book but also for being there whenever I seek for help.

******

I also dedicate this book to my mother Mary, for being a strong role model in my life. For her support, inspirations, reminding me to pray hard and motivating me when I feel like giving up. This dedication extends to my small brother Cyrus Lee for his great heart and his kindness.

******

Finally, I dedicate this Mind and Body Fitness Program, to you my friend, for making a choice to go for a 60-Day adventure with me. Let me know how this program has changed your life. Thank you!

Table of Contents

Introduction

Do you intend to attain a reasonable level of fitness? I suppose so because everybody needs it. Our reasons may differ widely – some of us consider the health benefits while others consider the aesthetic benefits – but in the end, fitness means something to most of us and that's probably the reason you're reading this right now.

The fitness goals most of us attempt to achieve are usually unrealized because:

- They may not mean so much to us.
- We may not set our goals right.
- We sabotage ourselves.

Regardless of whether you're just starting out or whether you've tried fitness programs before, you can follow this health and wellness mind and body fitness program to experience great results.

I have experienced the health benefits, personal satisfaction and peace of mind that come with this bikini beach bae mind and body wellness program and I would like to teach people the principles so they can duplicate it and benefit from it as well.

Contained in this book is a **workable 60-day challenge** and I believe that if you follow it diligently, you will arrive at a fruitful destination both in mind and body at the end of the period.

So are you ready to challenge yourself? Let's go!

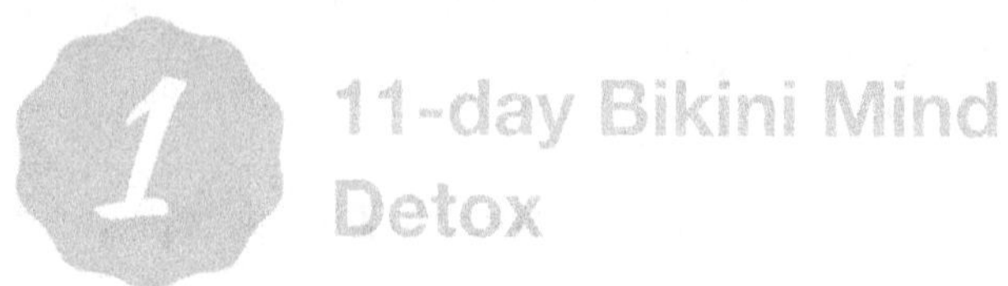

11-day Bikini Mind Detox

Before effecting any changes, including fitness goals, on the physical, we must make changes on the inside, on the mental side. This step is very critical to the success of any program. Many endeavors fail right from the get-go simply because the participant was not mentally prepped to go all the way.

So are you ready to go through this program effectively and come out a better, fitter person?

Just like a body detox program is used to rid the physical body of harmful substances and return it to a healthy, balanced condition, a mind detox can also be used to similar effect on the mental plane. While a mind detox will rid you of harmful, painful and misdirected thoughts and emotions, it can also help you start healthy habits that will be beneficial to you.

The emotional and behavioral aspects of a mind detox can help you to achieve the following things:

- A more focused mind.
- A calmer disposition.
- A better mood.

In order to expel all negative thoughts weighing you down, you have to start by taking some preparatory steps.

The following are steps you can practice alongside your step-by- step 11-day action points.

1- Put your thoughts on paper: writing your thoughts down on paper is one of the most effective techniques to get your mind fully detoxified.

Perform this step by writing down your exact stream of consciousness. The thoughts that come to mind, in their unbridled, uncut manner should be written on paper. You'll then be able to see the things that cloud your mind. As the days go by, watch which thoughts leave and which ones remain behind.

Work on the positive thoughts so they can come to fruition and forget about the negative ones.

2- Practice deep breathing: Breathing is mostly an unconscious activity and when we breathe, we most likely practice "surface breathing".

This is the process by which we breathe primarily by letting air enter and exit only our upper chest.

To reduce stressful thoughts and calm yourself deeply, breathe slowly, letting the air fill your whole diaphragm before exhaling. Do this at least 10 times.

3- Practice meditation: meditation is the practice of focusing your mind on only one particular object or thought in a bid to achieve a mentally clear and emotionally calm state.

This definition clarifies a lot about meditation especially for those who think it is just a time-wasting technique. The benefits of this age- long practice can be enjoyed by simply practicing it regularly.

Start by breathing deeply and finding a rhythm. As you relax, you can choose to close your eyes to avoid distractions. If you choose to open your eyes, stare ahead of you and try to let your eyes relax without focusing on any exact point.

After you have fully relaxed, you can focus on a thought, by visualizing it and using affirming words to build it in your mind.

Day 1 of 11: MIND EXAMINATION

Take a pen and a notebook and write down all the negative thoughts and feelings that you know are holding you back and burdening your day to day life.

ACTION STEP: find a calm place away from distractions (phone, children, spouses, computers and other digital devices).

Lie down flat or sit in your most comfortable position and begin to meditate.

During this meditation time, search in your mind for harmful thoughts about things, people around you or from your past that block you to move to a better healthy life.

When you're done, take your pen and note book and write down (identify) those negative thoughts. Note that you should never be in a hurry to complete this step!

Be patient with yourself. If you find 1 thing, don't worry, wait for another moment on this first day to re-do the mind meditation. If after the 2nd and 3rd trial, you still can't capture any harmful thoughts, wait for tomorrow – day 2 of 11.

I suggest you do this early in the morning when it's calm because at the end of the day, you might be very tired.

Continue with your mind examination and active search of all harmful and negative thoughts in your mind.

Find painful moments in your life from both your past and present. Add more things to your list.

Bleed into it; this is the basis of Mind Detox. And speak your thoughts as you write them down.

ACTION STEP: do 1 or 2 things from your list.

For example, if you wrote, "lack of physical exercise", then step out and go do a physical exercise e.g. running, walking, swimming for 30 to 45 minutes.

Finalize the listing and identification of all your harmful or negative thoughts and feelings. Make sure you totally empty your mind.

ACTION STEP: do 3 to 4 things from your list.

Write 10 things from your past life that you're grateful about. (Think about how all these things have molded you to be the person you're today).

Write 10 things in your present life that you're grateful about.

Write 10 things that you'll no longer tolerate or accept in your life.

Write 10 things or adventures that make you happy.

Name 10 people that inspire and motivate you in your daily life. They could be real or fictional.

DAY 9, 10 AND 11

Identify and list down what you want to become. Write down the changes you want in your body (Day 9), mind (Day 10), and spirit (Day 11). Keep listing the action steps that you need to apply in order to reach your goals and to become what you dream and aspire to become. Meditate and envision your future self and life.

2 7-day Mind Feeding and Nourishment

Your mindset is very important to how your life turns out. You can't be in control of many things, in fact, we're hardly ever in control of anything but how we're fully in control of how we react. It is how you react to the situations you're served that determines how well things will go. You're not guaranteed that you'll receive all the best of situations and experiences and talents but how will you react? With a brooding, complaining disposition or with a smiling, flexible one?

Do you know those people who always seem to be smiling no matter whether it's cloudy, depressingly raining or even when they just lost a job? They may seem annoying but they're having the best of life. This is not the reason they're always happy though; they're always happy because they're ready to move, bounce and spar with life. They have a good time because they've chosen to be happy in spite of their challenges. And if you look closely, you'll see that they always bounce back when they fall.

Do you want to be like that? Instead of remaining stuck because of a bad experience, would you rather move on with all the happiness and enthusiasm in the world?

If yes, then I'm glad to inform you that it can be done. You can become that happy person. You only need to make a mindshift to change your mindset. The moment you start doing this, you're already on your way.

There are certain words and phrases you can use to feed and nourish your mind. Slow, purposeful repetition of these words can help you effect the mindshift you so desperately need from a negative mental space to a positive one.

This is possible because words are very powerful to the point where they affect our reality. Whether you speak them to yourself, to others or to situations, words carry vibrations and it is better to use these vibrations for good instead of using them for evil or even letting them lie fallow.

Do you know that the vibrations carried by words operate on frequencies which influence the auras of human bodies? Thus, the spoken word, especially when repeated, can affect people – including ourselves – and the environment, thereby causing change to occur.

If you truly want to cause a mindshift in yourself, you can do it by consciously saying or chanting certain words, phrases and affirmations. This should be done with a few repetitions at least once a day.

It might be difficult or even counter-intuitive but negative situations can be surmounted by using the power of words for mind feeding and nourishment. Whenever you are ever faced with obstacles – and this will happen severally over the course of your life – you can choose to not speak negatively for you are only fueling the situation and making it thrive.

Instead, speak positively by affirming that your problems will be dealt with and that they will all turn out to be good in the end. This technique works by causing things to change in your favor and by giving you insight that you would not have been privy to with your mind in a negative space.

The following are words to repeat to yourself:
- Peace!
- Happiness!
- Tranquility!
- Abundance!

The following are short affirmations/phrases to repeat to yourself:

- Make it work!
- Don't worry, be happy!
- Keep calm and carry on!
- This too, shall pass!
- Everything is working for my good!
- Every little thing's gonna be alright!
- I will accept the things I cannot change!

The following are longer affirmations to repeat to yourself:

- May all beings everywhere be free and may the thoughts, words, and actions of my own life contribute in some way to that happiness and to that freedom for all.
- May health abound forever, may peace abound forever, may complete abundance abound forever, and may auspiciousness abound forever. Peace, Peace, Peace.

Note that you can create your own affirmations; reciting words that resonate with you and reflect your desires is very good for feeding and nourishing the mind.

The exercise you will undergo for the following seven days will consist of you focusing on a particular concept each day while repeating a personalized phrase or affirmation that applies to that concept.

DAY 1 OF 7: CHOICE

We have freedom of choice and you are where you are today because of the choices you've made. We become our own choices.

DAY 2 OF 7: HUNGER

Here we focus on what drives you to what you do.
What are you hungry for? Weight loss? A debt-free lifestyle? A flat tummy? Leadership?

DAY 3 OF 7: WORD

Both negative and positive words are very powerful. And in mind feeding, you decide where you want your words to direct you.

For example in this program, the goal is to have a healthy mind and body, so we focus on positive mind and feeding words.

DAY 4 OF 7: VISION

Through meditation, you can envision the kind of mind, body and spirit lifestyle you want and then start applying it in real life.

DAY 5 OF 7: PASSION

Passion is what drives you to achieve your goals.

Do you love what you're doing? Are you living your purpose?

DAY 6 OF 7: FAITH

You need to have a strong belief that what you're working for (weight loss, mindshift etc) is going to happen.
But know that faith has to be accompanied by action always.

DAY 7 OF 7: WORK

Yes you need to put in massive work in order to have massive results so start putting in that work right now.

3

Detoxification is simply the removal of harmful or toxic substances from the living human body. This could be physiological means including dieting and eating cleaner, healthier means or by strict medical processes including stomach pumping and drug therapy.

The medical techniques for detoxification are only used in cases where a person is in a critical state because of the amount of toxic substances in the body and because these substances have to be removed as quickly as possible. For this program, we are going to focus on the simple physiological detox where it is assumed that the person is in a stable okay condition and can simply assist the body in flushing toxic substances out naturally.

Detoxification is a process which has been practiced for centuries by certain cultures around the world. For instance, practitioners of Indian Ayurvedic and Chinese medicine have been using detoxification for many years to the benefit of many people.

So how exactly does a detox program work?

Detox is simply a process of helping and accelerating the body's natural tendency to clean and purify itself, the blood especially. The body does this mainly by expelling toxins through the liver but it also conducts detoxification through a few other organs including the kidney, the lungs, the skin and the lymphatic system.

Considering that we sometimes eat and drink too much junk – and this can go on for days or weeks at a time – it is important to practice detoxification regularly to help the body's overloaded systems to purify itself.

The following are a few ways that detoxification can assist the body in its bid to clean itself:

- Stimulating the liver to drive toxins from the body.
- Improving circulation of the blood.
- Resting the body organs through fasting.
- Promoting elimination of toxic substances through the intestines, kidneys, and skin.
- Refueling the body with healthy nutrients.

The basic idea of a true holistic detox program is to incorporate resting with the cleansing and nourishing of the body that occur from the inside out. If you can remove toxic substances from your body while simultaneously feeding on healthy, wholesome food, you will successfully detoxify your body and gain some useful things in the process.

The benefits of a successful detox include:
- Boosting of the immune system for improved protection against disease.
- Infusing participants with an increased energy that lasts throughout the day.
- A better ability to control cravings.
- A great way to curb food addiction.
- Giving the body essential micronutrients which it needs.
- Helping in stress management.

So how exactly do you know when the time has come for you to undergo detox?

General advice says that everybody should undergo detox at least once a year except children, nursing mothers, patients with tuberculosis, cancer or other degenerative diseases. If you fall into any of these excluded categories, you should ask consult your doctor or general healthcare practitioner to be sure that detoxifying is safe for you.

Since we live in modern times with multiple toxins from industries, automobiles and even from the food we eat, it has become critical to undergo detox and some tell-tale signs can be used as a form of alert to show you when it's time for your detox.

The "detox now" signs that everyone should look out for include:

- Unexplained fatigue.
- Irritated skin.
- Mental confusion.
- Low-grade infection.
- Puffy eyes or bags under the eyes.
- Bloating.
- Menstrual problems.

This bikini body detox runs for a period of 11 days because it takes time to clean the blood and so you should make every day count.

Note that going on a light diet is essential to detoxing. Do not see it as some form of punishment but as a way of cutting down on items that are difficult for your body to process. A little exercise should also be performed because it is good for cleansing out the body.

The exercise that follows consists of at least one activity coupled with a fruit or vegetable mix that should be drank each day.

The fruit mix should be made by blending and adding the fruits to 11⁄2 liters of water. The veggies should be diced neatly into a bowl and stirred to be eaten as a salad.

DAY 1 OF 11

- Drink at least 2 quarts of water a day.
- Perform deep breathing exercises.
- Fruit mix: lemon and orange.

DAY 2 OF 11

- Drink green tea or any other herbal teas like milk thistle and dandelion root. This will cleanse the liver and protect it.
- Fruit mix: Cucumber and apple.

DAY 3 OF 11

- Take in a lot of vitamin C. This is because glutathlone's production in the liver for expelling toxic substances is aided by vitamin C.
- Fruit mix: Lemon and lime.

DAY 4 OF 11

- Perform hydrotherapy. This can easily be done by taking a 5-minute hot shower. This shower is then to be followed by a 30-second cold shower. This hot and cold alternation should be done three times.
- Fruit mix: Beets and orange.

DAY 5 OF 11

- De-emphasize negative emotions by minimizing them and looking on the bright side while emphasizing positive emotions by dwelling on them.
- Veggie mix: beets and radish.

DAY 6 OF 11

- Attend a sauna and perform a full body routine. Ensure that you don't leave until you've broken out into a good sweat; this helps your body eliminate toxic substances via perspiration.
- Veggie mix: Cabbage and radish.

DAY 7 OF 11

- Focus on your lower limbs and detoxify any toxins nestled there. Do this by dry-brushing the skin on your feet. You can also visit a special foot spa or foot bathhouse so you can expel toxins from your feet professionally. At foot spas, the process is much easier because special brushes are used. (You can also get these brushes at natural products stores).
- Fruit mix: Grapefruit and apple.

DAY 8 OF 11

- Detoxify by getting into a little exercise. The most effective ones for a successful detox include jump-roping, yoga or any form of aerobics.
- Veggie mix: Cabbage and broccoli.

- Engage in a light system of Qi gong. Qi gong is a Chinese system of physical exercises and breathing control related to Tai chi. The Qi gong system involves exercises specially designed for detoxifying or cleansing. Do not let the name frighten you though, simple Qi gong exercises exist and can be done.
- Fruit and veggie mix: Spirulina and chlorella.

DAY 10 OF 11

- Practice inversion. Inversion is the simple physiological process that involves flipping the natural human posture or position. Simple, traditional positions include headstands, handstands, shoulder stands and a simple propping of the legs against a wall. Inversions stimulate the lymphatic system and help in purifying the blood.
- Fruit and veggie mix: Lemon and ginger.

DAY 11 OF 11

- Take a detox bath. This is a very powerful method and it has four major ingredients: Dead sea salts/Epsom salts (2 cups), baking soda (2 cups), freshly ground ginger (1 tablespoon) and therapeutic-grade essential oils (4 drops).

- Fruit and veggie mix: Seaweed salad, nori and dulse.

Substances to stay away from during detox: alcohol, tobacco, refined sugars, caffeine, high-mercury fish and non-organic fruits and vegetables.

4. 21-day Bikini Body Feeding

What you put into your body counts. And no, I'm not even talking about calories. The simple act of feeding yourself goes a long way to determine how healthy you are and how energetic you feel. This is why it is very important to eat clean. It is the key to a lot of healthy results just as the opposite – eating junk, is fraught with lots of health problems. And of course from experience, I know that for that fit body, eating healthy is essential!

Eating clean may be showing up a lot online and on social media but what does it really mean?

Eating clean simply means making a conscious effort to eat the best and healthiest options in each of the food groups while consuming less of junk food.

Eating clean is not about reducing your calories or food categories like carbohydrates or protein although this might happen when you begin to eat clean. Eating clean is more about watching what your food has come in contact with from the time it was grown till the time it lands on your plate.

To eat clean, you must begin to embrace foods like whole grains, fruits and vegetables along with healthy proteins and fats. Think of whole foods as "real foods" or foods so minimally processed, they are as close to their natural, organic state as possible.

Eating such foods as mentioned above is only half of the game as eating clean would not be eating clean if you continued to binge on junk and processed foods. The other half of eating clean involves cutting down on foods with refined components including refined grains, unhealthy fats, large portions of salt and sugar and any food containing additives and preservatives. Another category of food to avoid is food grown with pesticides for they are quite unhealthy and their effects might take long periods to manifest.

A good way to recognize an additive is by checking out the name as displayed on the food pack. If it's a long, technical- sounding name, it most likely is a synthetic ingredient added to flavor the food or prolong its shelf life.

Eating clean doesn't have to happen all at once; you can start slowly and take it one step at a time. For instance, you could start by leaving your processed food intake as is while increasing your fruit and vegetable intake.

Eating clean is not easy, especially with the sophisticated nature of modern food processing but with a little effort, it can be done. I did it successfully and so can you!

Since eating clean might not be so straightforward, so I have put together a few simple steps to help you begin your journey to clean eating in earnest.

1- Make the switch to whole grain.

Whole grains are so healthy, it's amazing that more people are not gobbling it up. Unprocessed whole grains are very close to their harvested state and this is very obvious in grains like oats and wild rice. While whole grain is good and some people make efforts to eat it, they are sometimes misled by labels on food packs.

Note that whole grain should be the first thing on the ingredient list – not an afterthought; the list should contain recognizable items and there should be minimal sugar or none at all.

Whole grains give you more fiber and antioxidants than you can get from refined grain and if you intend to lose weight and keep the weight off, whole grain is the way to go.

2- Cut down on sugar.

Added sugar is so ubiquitous in food products today, most people eat them all up without even knowing.

Too much sugar is responsible for such health problems as weight gain, diabetes and a host of others. Unfortunately, while the American Heart Association recommends a maximum of six teaspoons of sugar a day for women and nine teaspoons for men, the reality is that on average, Americans eat about 28 teaspoons a day.

To cut down on your sugar intake, drastically reduce soda, candy and desserts. Also look out for "healthy" foods that are still flooded with sugar.

This list includes cereal, tomato sauce and even yoghurt. Instead, eat more of organic foods with naturally-occurring sugars; they are healthier, and contain other essentials like protein and fiber, thereby ensuring that you're not getting just empty calories.

3- Increase your fruit and vegetable intake.

You might think you eat enough fruits and vegetables but the reality of the situation is that you're likely not getting as much as you need.

The Center for Disease Control and Prevention states that the number of Americans who don't eat enough fruit everyday stands at 76 percent. The number for those who don't eat enough vegetables is even worse, standing at a whopping 87 percent. Eating fruits and vegetables is very important since this healthy category of food can help reduce the risk of developing multiple chronic illnesses including type-2 diabetes, high blood pressure, heart disease, cancer and obesity.

Also, the fibers so abundantly found in organic fruits and vegetables balance the amount of good bacteria in your stomach and this can help reduce the risk for autoimmune diseases while fighting infections and pathogens.

4- Cut down on meat.

By including this tip, I do not by any means mean that you should go vegan – if you have no intention of doing so.

Although, the evidence continues to pile up that eating less meat is great for you and even the planet, you don't need to be a vegetarian to partake of the process of eating clean. But the fact is this, reducing the amount of meat you eat can reduce your risk of heart disease, seriously reduce your blood pressure and stabilize your weight. If you're worried about the effects on your body, rest assured, you're most likely getting far more than you need.

It is recommended that the average person ingest about 0.8 grams of protein per kilogram but instead Americans eat much higher and strangely enough, they can get all that protein from foods that are not meat. For the little meat you eat, make sure it hasn't been loaded with antibiotics; you get bonus points if you eat meat from live animals that ate the way they would have in the wild.

5- Lay off processed foods.

To be clear, food processing is a loose term; shady food manufacturers say this a lot but it actually is a fact.

For food to be eaten, it has to be transformed from its raw form by one or more processes. This means that the different forms of cooking are actually forms of food processing. To be clear, when we use the term, we mean "industrially processed foods loaded with sugars, salts, chemical additives and hydrogenated oils."

It's important to lay off processed foods as part of eating clean because the human body digests processed foods in a very different way from unprocessed foods.

This difference starts at the ease with which the food is digested and ends at the nutrients or toxic substances absorbed. One other good reason for cutting down on processed foods is the avoidance of substances like BPA (Bisphenol A) and other chemical substances used in cans and plastic receptacles used to store food.

6- Cut the salt too!

Sugar isn't the only great-tasting substance which is needed by humans but overused; salt is, too.

This is because salt is thrown into a lot of main dishes and convenience foods in a bid to make them taste better and sadly, a lot of Americans have become hooked on this spicy-tasting product.

The problem here really is sodium, which is the major component of salt and also a huge factor in high blood pressure. It is recommended, by the Institute of Medicine, that sodium intake should not exceed 2,300 milligrams a day. In fact, for people living with diabetes, high blood pressure and kidney disease, the sodium intake should not be more than 1,500 milligrams a day.

Clearly, cutting down on processed foods, as discussed above (in tip 5), will help in bringing down your salt intake. To make this tip work properly, especially for those who dread eating bland, unsalted meals, remember that while salt might be the major spice, it is not the only one. You can spice up your food with herbs, curry, vinegar, citrus and a whole range of flavoring substances, along with a little salt.

7- Remember that the environment needs to be protected too.

If eating clean were only good for you, that would be reason enough to try it, wouldn't it? But now that it is known that eating clean can also significantly help the state of the planet, isn't that even more of an incentive to watch what we eat?

Getting food, especially in all its modern glory, takes away a lot from the earth and it really doesn't have to be so. It is believed that the modern process of agriculture is responsible for as much as a third of all greenhouse gas emissions.

The meat industry is especially culpable because of what it takes to feed and rear the animals needed to give meat. For instance, in the rearing of animals like cows, goat and sheep, the digestion process and waste products released from these animals contain a very high level of methane, contributing to the huge carbon footprint being left on the planet.

The fishing industry is not far behind. Indiscriminate fishing in water bodies has led to depletion of many species of seafood and the gradual destruction of natural marine habitats.

Growing of crops too, takes its own toll as the huge number of artificial fertilizers coupled with herbicides and pesticides widely used to raise them are all leading to a decline in soil and water quality.

Where does eating clean come in?

The more fruits and vegetables you eat, cutting down on meat, the more you help, since meat- based diets require 3 times more water and 2.5 times more energy to produce.

If we cut down on meat, you automatically cut down on greenhouse emissions. You could also choose farm-fed seafood or seafood that has been fished in a sustainable manner. Even the little meat you eat should be grass-fed, if possible.

8- Include supplements as part of your daily meal plan.

I decided to tackle this last because over the years, I have come to believe that supplements are too important to be ignored.

I've also come to understand that people do not easily grasp this importance. Most people see supplements as medication for sick people and so as long as they feel fine, their natural reaction is "Why do I need to take anything?" Here's why.

Firstly, modern food processing methods are doing a good job of stripping your food of their natural nutrients. Yes, if you eat normal, you're eating a lot of fodder. And even if you eat clean, except you go 100 percent organic, your food is grown on soils with depleted nutrients and so do not have all you need to start with.

Add that to food that has been in transit for weeks or months and which will most likely be overcooked – because that's what we know – then you begin to see that your food is grossly inadequate.

Also realize that sometimes we can't help but skip meals and that stressed bodies and compromised immune systems need more than food to fix.

So please, I encourage you to go for food supplements; they'll do your body a whole lot of good and the results will be clear to see.

Practical exercise

The following exercise in table format gives you a brief description of foods you can eat on your 21-day bikini body challenge.

	MEALS		
DAY	**Breakfast**	**Lunch**	**Dinner**
DAY 1	Avocado-egg toast	Tuna and white bean spinach salad	Brown rice with coconut-shallot sauce and fish
DAY 2	Plain Greek yogurt	Veggie sandwich	Spaghetti squash with meatballs
DAY 3	Toast whole-grain bread with peanut butter	Toast whole-grain bread with peanut butter	Brown rice with Brussels sprouts and salmon

DAY	Breakfast	Lunch	Dinner
DAY 4	Strawberry banana smoothie	Chickpea & veggie salad	Chicken and Quinoa
DAY 5	Slow cooker creamy almond oatmeal	Vegetable soup	Baked sweet potato, seared pork chops and roasted cabbage with Mustard-chive vinaigrette
DAY 6	Roasted, unsalted almonds or peanuts and a Green smoothie	A bowl of veggie-quinoa with Hummus dressing	Peanut-tofu cabbage wraps
DAY 7	Cherry chocolate chip pancakes	Bean and Barley soup	Shrimp and spiced black beans

DAY	Breakfast	Lunch	Dinner
DAY 8	Veggie scramble	Tuna and white bean spinach salad	Bean and Barley soup
DAY 9	Plain Greek yogurt	Veggie sandwich	Quinoa and chicken with steamed asparagus
DAY 10	Toasted whole-grain bread, peanut butter and a banana	Chickpea and vegetable salad	Roast pork, asparagus and cherry tomato bowl
DAY 11	Plain Greek yogurt	Vegetable salad	Roast chicken and fennel
DAY 12	Avocado-egg toast	Squash and red lentil curry	Poached cod and green beans with pesto
DAY 13	Plain Greek yogurt	Chickpea and vegetable salad	Squash and red lentil curry

DAY	Breakfast	Lunch	Dinner
DAY 14	Quinoa breakfast cereal	Avocado-egg toast with garden salad	Roasted beet salad with feta, pistachios and tangerine
DAY 15	Pumpkin spice bread with walnut butter	Chile- marinated skirt stake	Brown rice and five-spice chicken with Clementine
DAY 16	Overnight French toast casserole	Quinoa- stuffed delicata squash	Sausage, cabbage and root vegetable soup
DAY 17	Cherry chocolate chip pancakes	Shrimp piccata with zucchini noodles	Poached cod and green beans with pesto
DAY 18	Pumpkin smoothie	Brussels sprouts salad with chicken	Vegetable soup

DAY	Breakfast	Lunch	Dinner
DAY 19	Quinoa breakfast cereal	Spinach and roasted beet salad	Baked chicken fingers
DAY 20	Sliced fruit with walnut butter	Cobb salad	Slow cooker balsamic chicken with brown rice
DAY 21	Pumpkin spice bread	Spinach and bean burrito wrap	Turkey burgers with sun dried tomatoes and feta cheese

7-day Body and Mind Weeding

I am sure the program is going well for you so far. If you've followed the previous challenges dedicatedly, you're very close to your goals of physical, mental and spiritual fitness. But at the same time, you're at that critical place where negative thoughts can creep up on you and overturn the gains you've made in the past few weeks.

This is entirely normal. I mean, you've gone through some great disciplinary actions to bridle your cravings and it's only natural for them to fight back. Whether you win or lose this battle is critical to whether you will be able to take this challenge to the very end and whether you will be able to sustain it after the program is over.

So do you want to win or lose?

You'll need to go through the previous challenges and take stock. Which ones were you brilliant at? Which ones could you have done better at? You need to keep the positive thoughts you've had about yourself and your ability to go through with this while weeding out any negative thoughts or habits that may be trying to derail you on the road to achieving your mental, physical and spiritual fitness.

All of this is important because fitness starts with the mind. A clear, positive mind will spur you to greater exploits than you could ever accomplish with just physical strengths.

Over the course of the next 7 days, you're going to weed your mind of any dangerous, negative thoughts that might have crept in or even been there all along.

DAY 1 OF 7: understand how powerful negative thinking is.

Since we often do not realize the power of our minds, it's understandable that we let negative thoughts run through them regularly. Our minds strongly influence us on a subconscious level that is difficult to notice and so it is important to watch what enters it.

Negative thinking consists of doubts and fears that only paralyze the person; it also causes bad things to go unchecked. If you understand that thinking these thoughts only encourages them to happen, you'll be more aware of keeping your thoughts in check.

DAY 2 AND 3 OF 7: convert negativity into positivity.

Today, you have to work on your negative thoughts now that you're aware of their power. Watch out for when these thoughts come along and instead of affirming them or focusing on them, instead look at the other side – the positive side. For instance, instead of thinking how it could go wrong, think how it could go right. And if something eventually goes bad, think about the silver lining in the clouds.

DAY 4 AND 5 OF 7: speak positively.

You might have heard this advice severally and might have ascribed it to one of these "new age teachings." But have you tried it? What harm could possibly come to you from trying it out? Whether you've heard about it previously or not, speaking positively is a powerful tool that works with the power of the mind. When you say things, they happen. Situations bend. You are inspired and challenged to play your part in making things happen. Words and thoughts have a complimentary relationship, and while it may be difficult to just start thinking positively – especially if your mind is filled with weeds – you can jumpstart the process by saying positive words and affirmations. Just say it, over and over and in due time, thinking positively will become second nature to you.

DAY 6 OF 7: distance yourself from negativity.

Our surroundings affect us heavily and sometimes we cannot surmount the power of a negative place. But there is one thing we can do when we are severely threatened by the power of a negative place or people – we can walk away.

If you try too hard to associate with negative friends or live in a house or even town that brings you too much trauma, you might be overcome in the end. There's no shame in moving away, no shame in losing toxic friends. You don't lose the battle by walking away. In fact, if walking away is the only way to win, why not?

DAY 7 OF 7: start doing.

While negative thoughts might try to block you from doing the things important to you by letting you believe they cannot be done, realize that it's all in your head and go out and start doing!

When you put your all into your actions and eventually accomplish your objectives even with your doubts around you, it becomes evidence that you are far more capable than you thought and that negative thoughts are just hindrances.

This step can get you to start weeding out negative thoughts more actively and effectively.

As this program draws to a close, I am glad to announce to you that you are pretty much that mentally and physically person you've always wanted to be. The essence of this last stretch of the program is to get you to actually enjoy the process of mental and physical fitness.

You must have seen tangible results by now, you must have also felt some of the goodness that comes with knowing that you're doing well for yourself. But have you enjoyed the journey so far? Have you had fun with it or has this been a case of "work, work and more work" to you?

Embracing this process as a regular part of you is critical to its success. If you've gone round performing this program grudgingly, you can start now to smile, for the benefits are all yours and believe me, it only gets easier as you go along.

In addition to your practical physical and mental exercises, you should go ahead and perform the activities that you enjoy doing, as long as they do not take away the gains of the past few weeks. For instance, jumping back to binge on alcohol or sugary desserts is a bad idea that will only erase a lot of the work you've put in. There's nothing wrong with a treat every now and then but making them regulars defeats the whole purpose. Besides, they are called treats for a reason.

So what can you do to get yourself to relax these few days and live that bikini beach bae life?

It really is up to you! But here are a few tips for living it up as you round up:

DAY 1 OF 3: have fun!

It is imperative that you have fun, if not during the program exercises themselves, then before and after you've completed them. If you have any hobbies you've been nursing, feel free to explore them now! If there are any passions you may have neglected, feel free to re-ignite the flame! Go out of your comfort zone and just try something new; it helps.

In my case, I did a few things I love to do. I went to the beach and I also participated in a beautiful photoshoot. It was incredibly fun.

So today, your job is really simple. Find what you've always wanted to do and just do it!

DAY 2 OF 3: assess yourself!

When you picked up this book and chose to follow this program, you must have had some expectations. Not only of the book but of yourself. Did you have any specific mental and physical goals that you hoped to meet? I'm sure you did.

Regardless of whether you wrote these expectations down or stored them mentally, they were right there with you and probably still are. Now bring these objectives up and ask yourself, at this point, what have you achieved? When you've done this, I'm sure you'll have a lot to smile about.

DAY 3 OF 3: prepare to stay in shape!

As your program ends today, realize one thing, you have to make this a part of your life. Eating clean, exercising your body, feeding your mind and all the other things you've learned do not end after today. Of course, they may not be as intense as during this 60-day period but they have to go on in lighter versions.

If you like what you've become, continue to live healthy!

Conclusion

wrote this book because I truly believe it will be unfair to keep all I learned during my fitness journey to myself. I have discovered that true fitness starts from inside. Consequently, most people jump into fitness programs and either gain no results or are unable to maintain them.

With all you've learned from the 60-day bikini beach bae mind and body program, your case will surely be different. As long as you keep up with this program and incorporate "healthiness" into your lifestyle, you will continue to enjoy the benefits of a fit body and an alert mind.

I wish you all the very best as you start your life as the newfound you.

Good luck!